Busy Thoughts Before Bed

Notebook Journal for those who can't sleep

Scripture taken from the King James Version is marked with (KJV) at the end of a quotation.

Scripture taken from New International Version Bible is marked with (NIV) on the end of a quotation.

Books are available at special discounts for bulk orders.

Book design and artwork done by Passionate Portraits

www.passionateportraitsweb.com

Printed in the United States of America

10 9 8 7 6 5 4 3 2 1

I dedicate this book to all those people struggling to find rest.

Other Titles by T. S. Thompson

Busy Thoughts Before Bed

This book belongs to:

Bible Verses
on Resting

Psalm 127:2 (KJV)
It is vain for you to rise up early, to sit up late, to eat the bread of sorrows: for so he giveth his beloved sleep.

> Sometimes we all think "the harder I work, the better things should be." But God just called you His beloved! God wants us to trust in Him, to the point of resting in Him. This verse is saying that rising early to work and staying up late to work is not His plan for you. He gives us sleep, so receive it, and rest.

Matthew 11:28 (NIV)
Come to me, all you who are weary and burdened, and I will give you rest.

> Here is an invitation from God to come to Him, those who are weary and burdened. Then He will give you rest. But the key here is to come to Him. Carrying your own burdens makes you weary and results in a lack of rest. I mean, how can you rest while carrying such a load? Receive His invitation and go to Him. He has promised when you come to Him, weary and burdened, He will give you rest.

Exodus 33:14 (KJV)
And he said, My presence shall go with thee, and I will give thee rest.

Part of difficulty falling asleep at night is feeling like you are all alone in whatever is keeping you up. But God is saying He goes with you. You are not alone. His presence is with you, you can rest in Him.

Psalm 91:1 (NIV)
Whoever dwells in the shelter of the Most High will rest in the shadow of the Almighty

This is my favorite Psalm and I read it often during difficult times. This part of the psalm is saying that those who seek God and His shelter will also rest in His shadow. I love how this verse refers to Him here as almighty. He is powerful and strong guarding over us.

Psalm 4:8 (NIV)
In peace I will lie down and sleep, for you alone, Lord, make me dwell in safety.

This is such a comforting verse to say before bed. Knowing that the Lord watches over me and keeps me safe while I sleep helps me rest.

Proverbs 3:24 (NIV)
When you lie down, you will not be afraid; when you lie down, your sleep will be sweet.

Isn't that beautiful? When we lie down and allow ourselves to rest, the Lord is saying our sleep will be sweet. This is the verse I like to read right before I go to sleep, so my thoughts are on the Word and not all the other crap rolling around in my head.

Bible Verses
on Worry

Philippians 4:6-7 (NIV)
Do not be anxious about anything, but in every situation, by prayer and petition, with thanksgiving, present your requests to God. And the peace of God, which transcends all understanding, will guard your hearts and your minds in Christ Jesus.

> God is very clear here that we are not to worry about anything. He did not record any exceptions. Then He instructs us what to do when we feel anxious. We are to pray. He even tells us how to pray. We are to petition our request to God with thanksgiving. Meaning, we approach God with our troubles with thanksgiving in our hearts because God told us that whatever we ask for, believe that we receive it and we shall have it. So we go knowing He has answered us. That is why we have thanksgiving. Here is the beautiful part. God promises us peace beyond our understanding because Jesus keeps our hearts and minds in Him! This truth is why there is never a reason to be anxious.

Psalm 55:22 (KJV)
Cast thy burden upon the Lord, and he shall sustain thee: he shall never suffer the righteous to be moved.

> In this verse I learned that if I haven't cast my burdens on the Lord, that I am the one trying to sustain myself. But when I cast them to God, meaning discard them and no longer have them, I allow God to sustain me. If I am still worrying, then I have not cast. The point

of casting is to get rid of it.

1 Peter 5:7 (KJV)

Casting all your care upon him; for he careth for you.

> Why does God want us to cast our cares to Him?
> Because He cares. He loves us beyond our comprehension. Trust Him.

2 Corinthians 10:5 (KJV)

Casting down imaginations, and every high thing that exalteth itself against the knowledge of God, and bringing into captivity every thought to the obedience of Christ;

> All of our worries come from what we are thinking about; the "what if this happens" or "what if that happens." We let our mind play out all sorts of scenarios that never happen. God says we can cast down those thoughts. Any thought that comes against the word of God; we can bring it into the captivity of Christ. So when bad thoughts enter your mind, cast them out and instead focus your thoughts on what the Word says.

John 14:27 (KJV)

Peace I leave with you, my peace I give unto you: not as the world giveth, give I unto you. Let not your heart be troubled, neither let it be afraid.

> Here is another verse on letting His peace cover your hearts. Do not let yourself worry over things and do not be fearful. Remember Jesus has overcome the world. Everything in this world is under His feet. He has overcome it. He is bigger than your problems. Have peace in that.

Jeremiah 32:17 (KJV)

Ah Lord God! behold, thou hast made the heaven and the earth by thy great power and stretched out arm, and there is nothing too hard for thee:

> Just in case you feel that what you are going through is too much for God, rest in the fact that he was clear that nothing is too hard for Him. Magnify God over your problems. Learn to see God as the victory over them.

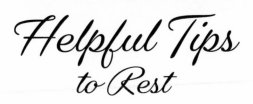

Helpful Tips
to Rest

Tip #1

Getting exercise during the day is a great way to help your body rest at night. I have found that if I exercise in the evening I stay pumped up for too long, making it harder to sleep. But a good morning or afternoon workout is great for the body. Even if you can't physically do much, a 30-minute walk will still benefit you.

Tip #2

I have found that limiting caffeine past 4 pm has also helped me to go to bed sooner rather than later.

Tip #3

I try not to eat anything heavy an hour before bedtime. I find an apple is a good snack before bed. It fills me up, but it's not heavy and digests easy. Plus the skin has a lot of fiber and helps keep you regular.

Tip #4

It is recommended to stop screen time an hour before bed. This is because of the blue light that comes from devices like phones, TV, and laptops. Blue light suppresses the production of melatonin, a hormone that regulates our sleep. Some newer phones have a night mode where it reduces blue light. You can also purchase amber glasses. These blue blocker glasses block the blue light from your eyes. Electronics may stimulate you despite blocking the blue light, so it is still a good practice to shut them off an hour before bed.

Tip #5

I recommend reading before bed as it is a relaxing alternative to watching TV or videos on your phone. Reading helps take my mind off of things I need to do or think about. Typically I read until my eyes feel heavy. Then I turn out my light and only focus on the book and nothing in my life that would prevent me from falling asleep.

Tip #6

I love a cup of Chamomile with Lavender tea before bed. It smells amazing, and it relaxes me for sleep. I dislike how Chamomile tastes by itself and the Lavender adds a sweet natural flavor so I do not need to add any honey. I drink my tea while reading for a good double combo to help me sleep.

Tip #7

Because I drink tea before bed, I have to get up to use the restroom once or twice a night. My rule is to not think about anything during this bathroom trip. If I let a thought come in and dwell on it, there's a high probability I won't be able to go back to sleep.

Tip #8

In difficult scenarios of travel or a snoring partner, there are helpful background noise apps for your phone. These soothing sounds of crickets or waves can be useful when sleep is harder than normal.

Tip #9

The biggest tip is to learn how to clear your busy mind before bedtime. That is why I created this journal. Keep it by your bed and when thoughts of stress creep in, write those thoughts down, and pray over them. If your mind is racing with things you need to remember to do, write them down and check off when you complete them another day. If you are a creative person like me and get a thought of inspiration right before bed, write it down so you can finish working on it tomorrow. This way you can rest knowing your busy thoughts are over there written in your journal and you can let your mind shut off for the night.

Date: _____   Time: _____

To do list	*Creative Ideas*
☐	
☐	
☐	
☐	
☐	
☐	
☐	
☐	
☐	
☐	

Stressful Thoughts

_____

_____

_____

_____

_____

Date: Time:

To do list	*Creative Ideas*
☐	
☐	
☐	
☐	
☐	
☐	
☐	
☐	
☐	
☐	

Stressful Thoughts

Date: Time:

To do list	Creative Ideas
☐	
☐	
☐	
☐	
☐	
☐	
☐	
☐	
☐	
☐	

Stressful Thoughts

Date: Time:

To do list	Creative Ideas
☐	
☐	
☐	
☐	
☐	
☐	
☐	
☐	
☐	
☐	

Stressful Thoughts

Date: Time:

To do list	∽ Creative Ideas ∾
☐	
☐	
☐	
☐	
☐	
☐	
☐	
☐	
☐	
☐	

∽ Stressful Thoughts ∾

To do list	Creative Ideas
☐	
☐	
☐	
☐	
☐	
☐	
☐	
☐	
☐	
☐	

Stressful Thoughts

Date: Time:

To do list | Creative Ideas

- [ ]
- [ ]
- [ ]
- [ ]
- [ ]
- [ ]
- [ ]
- [ ]
- [ ]
- [ ]

Stressful Thoughts

Date: Time:

To do list	Creative Ideas
☐	
☐	
☐	
☐	
☐	
☐	
☐	
☐	
☐	
☐	

Stressful Thoughts

Date: _____   Time: _____

To do list	∽ Creative Ideas ∽
☐	
☐	
☐	
☐	
☐	
☐	
☐	
☐	
☐	
☐	

∽ Stressful Thoughts ∽

Date: Time:

To do list	Creative Ideas
☐	
☐	
☐	
☐	
☐	
☐	
☐	
☐	
☐	
☐	

Stressful Thoughts

Date: Time:

To do list	Creative Ideas
☐	
☐	
☐	
☐	
☐	
☐	
☐	
☐	
☐	
☐	

Stressful Thoughts

Date: _____   Time: _____

To do list	Creative Ideas
☐	
☐	
☐	
☐	
☐	
☐	
☐	
☐	
☐	
☐	

Stressful Thoughts

_____

_____

_____

_____

_____

_____

Date: Time:

To do list	Creative Ideas
☐	
☐	
☐	
☐	
☐	
☐	
☐	
☐	
☐	
☐	

Stressful Thoughts

To do list

☐

☐

☐

☐

☐

☐

☐

☐

☐

☐

∽ Creative Ideas ∽

∽ Stressful Thoughts ∽

Date: Time:

To do list	∽ Creative Ideas ∽
☐	
☐	
☐	
☐	
☐	
☐	
☐	
☐	
☐	
☐	

∽ Stressful Thoughts ∽

Date: Time:

To do list	∽Creative Ideas∼
☐	
☐	
☐	
☐	
☐	
☐	
☐	
☐	
☐	
☐	

∽Stressful Thoughts∼

Date: Time:

To do list	Creative Ideas
☐	
☐	
☐	
☐	
☐	
☐	
☐	
☐	
☐	
☐	

Stressful Thoughts

Date: Time:

To do list	Creative Ideas
☐	
☐	
☐	
☐	
☐	
☐	
☐	
☐	
☐	
☐	

Stressful Thoughts

Date: Time:

To do list	❦ Creative Ideas ❧
☐	
☐	
☐	
☐	
☐	
☐	
☐	
☐	
☐	
☐	

❦ Stressful Thoughts ❧

Date: Time:

To do list	*Creative Ideas*
☐	
☐	
☐	
☐	
☐	
☐	
☐	
☐	
☐	
☐	

Stressful Thoughts

Date: Time:

To do list	Creative Ideas
☐	
☐	
☐	
☐	
☐	
☐	
☐	
☐	
☐	
☐	

Stressful Thoughts

Date: Time:

To do list	∽ Creative Ideas ∾
☐	
☐	
☐	
☐	
☐	
☐	
☐	
☐	
☐	
☐	

∽ Stressful Thoughts ∾

Date: _____   Time: _____

To do list	*Creative Ideas*
☐	
☐	
☐	
☐	
☐	
☐	
☐	
☐	
☐	
☐	

Stressful Thoughts

Date: Time:

To do list | *Creative Ideas*

- [ ]
- [ ]
- [ ]
- [ ]
- [ ]
- [ ]
- [ ]
- [ ]
- [ ]
- [ ]

Stressful Thoughts

Date: Time:

To do list	Creative Ideas
☐	
☐	
☐	
☐	
☐	
☐	
☐	
☐	
☐	
☐	

Stressful Thoughts

Date: Time:

To do list	Creative Ideas
☐	
☐	
☐	
☐	
☐	
☐	
☐	
☐	
☐	
☐	

Stressful Thoughts

Date: Time:

To do list	Creative Ideas
☐	
☐	
☐	
☐	
☐	
☐	
☐	
☐	
☐	
☐	

Stressful Thoughts

Date: Time:

To do list	Creative Ideas
☐	
☐	
☐	
☐	
☐	
☐	
☐	
☐	
☐	
☐	

Stressful Thoughts

Date: Time:

To do list	Creative Ideas
☐	
☐	
☐	
☐	
☐	
☐	
☐	
☐	
☐	
☐	

Stressful Thoughts

To do list

Creative Ideas

- [ ]
- [ ]
- [ ]
- [ ]
- [ ]
- [ ]
- [ ]
- [ ]
- [ ]
- [ ]

Stressful Thoughts

Date: Time:

To do list	*Creative Ideas*
☐	
☐	
☐	
☐	
☐	
☐	
☐	
☐	
☐	
☐	

Stressful Thoughts

Date: _____   Time: _____

To do list	Creative Ideas
☐	
☐	
☐	
☐	
☐	
☐	
☐	
☐	
☐	
☐	

Stressful Thoughts

Date: _____   Time: _____

To do list	Creative Ideas
☐	
☐	
☐	
☐	
☐	
☐	
☐	
☐	
☐	
☐	

Stressful Thoughts

Date: Time:

To do list	*Creative Ideas*
☐	
☐	
☐	
☐	
☐	
☐	
☐	
☐	
☐	
☐	

Stressful Thoughts

To do list · Creative Ideas ·

- [ ]
- [ ]
- [ ]
- [ ]
- [ ]
- [ ]
- [ ]
- [ ]
- [ ]
- [ ]

· Stressful Thoughts ·

Date: Time:

To do list	*Creative Ideas*
☐	
☐	
☐	
☐	
☐	
☐	
☐	
☐	
☐	
☐	

Stressful Thoughts

Date: Time:

To do list	Creative Ideas
☐	
☐	
☐	
☐	
☐	
☐	
☐	
☐	
☐	
☐	

Stressful Thoughts

Date: Time:

To do list	*Creative Ideas*
☐	
☐	
☐	
☐	
☐	
☐	
☐	
☐	
☐	
☐	

Stressful Thoughts

Date: _____   Time: _____

To do list	Creative Ideas
☐	
☐	
☐	
☐	
☐	
☐	
☐	
☐	
☐	
☐	

Stressful Thoughts

Date: Time:

To do list	*Creative Ideas*
☐	
☐	
☐	
☐	
☐	
☐	
☐	
☐	
☐	
☐	

Stressful Thoughts

Date: _____   Time: _____

To do list	Creative Ideas
☐	
☐	
☐	
☐	
☐	
☐	
☐	
☐	
☐	
☐	

Stressful Thoughts

Date: _____   Time: _____

To do list	*Creative Ideas*
☐	
☐	
☐	
☐	
☐	
☐	
☐	
☐	
☐	
☐	

Stressful Thoughts

Date: Time:

To do list	Creative Ideas
☐	
☐	
☐	
☐	
☐	
☐	
☐	
☐	
☐	
☐	

Stressful Thoughts

Date: _____   Time: _____

To do list	Creative Ideas
☐	
☐	
☐	
☐	
☐	
☐	
☐	
☐	
☐	
☐	

Stressful Thoughts

_____

_____

_____

_____

_____

_____

Date: Time:

To do list	Creative Ideas
☐	
☐	
☐	
☐	
☐	
☐	
☐	
☐	
☐	
☐	

Stressful Thoughts

Date: _____   Time: _____

To do list	Creative Ideas
☐	_____
	_____
☐	_____
	_____
☐	_____
	_____
☐	_____
	_____
☐	_____
	_____
☐	_____
	_____
☐	_____
	_____
☐	_____
	_____
☐	_____
	_____
☐	_____

Stressful Thoughts

_____

_____

_____

_____

_____

_____

Date: Time:

To do list	Creative Ideas
☐	
☐	
☐	
☐	
☐	
☐	
☐	
☐	
☐	
☐	

Stressful Thoughts

Date: Time:

To do list	*Creative Ideas*
☐	
☐	
☐	
☐	
☐	
☐	
☐	
☐	
☐	
☐	

Stressful Thoughts

Date: Time:

To do list

Creative Ideas

- [ ]
- [ ]
- [ ]
- [ ]
- [ ]
- [ ]
- [ ]
- [ ]
- [ ]
- [ ]

Stressful Thoughts

Date: Time:

To do list	Creative Ideas
☐	
☐	
☐	
☐	
☐	
☐	
☐	
☐	
☐	
☐	

Stressful Thoughts

Date: Time:

To do list	_Creative Ideas_
☐	
☐	
☐	
☐	
☐	
☐	
☐	
☐	
☐	
☐	

Stressful Thoughts

Date: _____   Time: _____

To do list	Creative Ideas
☐	
☐	
☐	
☐	
☐	
☐	
☐	
☐	
☐	
☐	

Stressful Thoughts

To do list

☐

☐

☐

☐

☐

☐

☐

☐

☐

☐

Creative Ideas

Stressful Thoughts

Date: Time:

To do list	Creative Ideas
☐	
☐	
☐	
☐	
☐	
☐	
☐	
☐	
☐	
☐	

Stressful Thoughts

Date: Time:

To do list	⌒ Creative Ideas ⌒
☐	
☐	
☐	
☐	
☐	
☐	
☐	
☐	
☐	
☐	

⌒ Stressful Thoughts ⌒

Date: Time:

To do list	Creative Ideas
☐	
☐	
☐	
☐	
☐	
☐	
☐	
☐	
☐	
☐	

Stressful Thoughts

To do list

☐

☐

☐

☐

☐

☐

☐

☐

☐

☐

∽ Creative Ideas ∾

∽ Stressful Thoughts ∾

Date: Time:

To do list

□

□

□

□

□

□

□

□

□

□

᥯ Creative Ideas ᥯

᥯ Stressful Thoughts ᥯

To do list	Creative Ideas
☐	
☐	
☐	
☐	
☐	
☐	
☐	
☐	
☐	
☐	

Stressful Thoughts

Date: _____   Time: _____

To do list	Creative Ideas
☐	
☐	
☐	
☐	
☐	
☐	
☐	
☐	
☐	
☐	

Stressful Thoughts

Date: _____   Time: _____

To do list	Creative Ideas
☐	
☐	
☐	
☐	
☐	
☐	
☐	
☐	
☐	
☐	

Stressful Thoughts

To do list   *Creative Ideas*

- [ ]
- [ ]
- [ ]
- [ ]
- [ ]
- [ ]
- [ ]
- [ ]
- [ ]
- [ ]

Stressful Thoughts

Date: Time:

To do list	~ Creative Ideas ~
☐	
☐	
☐	
☐	
☐	
☐	
☐	
☐	
☐	
☐	

~ Stressful Thoughts ~

Date: Time:

To do list   *Creative Ideas*

☐

☐

☐

☐

☐

☐

☐

☐

☐

☐

Stressful Thoughts

Date: _____   Time: _____

To do list	Creative Ideas
☐	_____
	_____
☐	_____
	_____
☐	_____
	_____
☐	_____
	_____
☐	_____
	_____
☐	_____
	_____
☐	_____
	_____
☐	_____
	_____
☐	_____
	_____
☐	_____

Stressful Thoughts

_____

_____

_____

_____

_____

_____

Date: _____   Time: _____

To do list	Creative Ideas
☐	
☐	
☐	
☐	
☐	
☐	
☐	
☐	
☐	
☐	

Stressful Thoughts

Date: Time:

To do list	Creative Ideas
☐	
☐	
☐	
☐	
☐	
☐	
☐	
☐	
☐	
☐	

Stressful Thoughts

Date: Time:

To do list	*Creative Ideas*
☐	
☐	
☐	
☐	
☐	
☐	
☐	
☐	
☐	
☐	

Stressful Thoughts

Date: Time:

To do list   Creative Ideas

- [ ]
- [ ]
- [ ]
- [ ]
- [ ]
- [ ]
- [ ]
- [ ]
- [ ]
- [ ]

Stressful Thoughts

Date: Time:

To do list	Creative Ideas
☐	_____
	_____
☐	_____
	_____
☐	_____
	_____
☐	_____
	_____
☐	_____
	_____
☐	_____
	_____
☐	_____
	_____
☐	_____
	_____
☐	_____
	_____
☐	_____

Stressful Thoughts

_____
_____
_____
_____
_____

Date: Time:

To do list	Creative Ideas
☐	
☐	
☐	
☐	
☐	
☐	
☐	
☐	
☐	
☐	

Stressful Thoughts

Date: _____   Time: _____

To do list	Creative Ideas
☐	
☐	
☐	
☐	
☐	
☐	
☐	
☐	
☐	
☐	

Stressful Thoughts

Date: Time:

To do list	Creative Ideas
☐	
☐	
☐	
☐	
☐	
☐	
☐	
☐	
☐	
☐	

Stressful Thoughts

Date: Time:

To do list	∾ Creative Ideas ∾
☐	
☐	
☐	
☐	
☐	
☐	
☐	
☐	
☐	
☐	

∾ Stressful Thoughts ∾

Date: Time:

To do list	ᴏ Creative Ideas ᴏ
☐	
☐	
☐	
☐	
☐	
☐	
☐	
☐	
☐	
☐	

ᴏ Stressful Thoughts ᴏ

To do list | Creative Ideas

- [ ]
- [ ]
- [ ]
- [ ]
- [ ]
- [ ]
- [ ]
- [ ]
- [ ]
- [ ]

Stressful Thoughts

Date: Time:

To do list

☐

☐

☐

☐

☐

☐

☐

☐

☐

☐

∽ Creative Ideas ∽

∽ Stressful Thoughts ∽

Date: _____   Time: _____

To do list	Creative Ideas
☐	
☐	
☐	
☐	
☐	
☐	
☐	
☐	
☐	
☐	

Stressful Thoughts

_____

_____

_____

_____

_____

Date: _____   Time: _____

To do list	∽Creative Ideas∾
☐	
☐	
☐	
☐	
☐	
☐	
☐	
☐	
☐	
☐	

∽Stressful Thoughts∾

Date: Time:

To do list	*Creative Ideas*
☐	
☐	
☐	
☐	
☐	
☐	
☐	
☐	
☐	
☐	

Stressful Thoughts

Date: Time:

To do list	Creative Ideas
☐	
☐	
☐	
☐	
☐	
☐	
☐	
☐	
☐	
☐	

Stressful Thoughts

Date: Time:

To do list | Creative Ideas

- ☐
- ☐
- ☐
- ☐
- ☐
- ☐
- ☐
- ☐
- ☐
- ☐

Stressful Thoughts

Date: Time:

To do list	Creative Ideas
☐	
☐	
☐	
☐	
☐	
☐	
☐	
☐	
☐	
☐	

Stressful Thoughts

Date: _____   Time: _____

To do list	*Creative Ideas*
☐	_____
	_____
☐	_____
	_____
☐	_____
	_____
☐	_____
	_____
☐	_____
	_____
☐	_____
	_____
☐	_____
	_____
☐	_____
	_____
☐	_____
	_____
☐	_____

Stressful Thoughts

_____

_____

_____

_____

_____

Date: Time:

To do list	Creative Ideas
☐	
☐	
☐	
☐	
☐	
☐	
☐	
☐	
☐	
☐	

Stressful Thoughts

Date: Time:

To do list	Creative Ideas
☐	
☐	
☐	
☐	
☐	
☐	
☐	
☐	
☐	
☐	

Stressful Thoughts

Date: Time:

To do list	Creative Ideas
☐	
☐	
☐	
☐	
☐	
☐	
☐	
☐	
☐	
☐	

Stressful Thoughts

Date: Time:

To do list	Creative Ideas
☐	
☐	
☐	
☐	
☐	
☐	
☐	
☐	
☐	
☐	

Stressful Thoughts

Date: Time:

To do list	*Creative Ideas*
☐	
☐	
☐	
☐	
☐	
☐	
☐	
☐	
☐	
☐	

Stressful Thoughts

_____

_____

_____

_____

_____

_____

Date: Time:

To do list	Creative Ideas
☐	
☐	
☐	
☐	
☐	
☐	
☐	
☐	
☐	
☐	

Stressful Thoughts

Date: Time:

To do list	~Creative Ideas~
☐	
☐	
☐	
☐	
☐	
☐	
☐	
☐	
☐	
☐	

~Stressful Thoughts~

Date: _____   Time: _____

To do list	ᦉ Creative Ideas ᦉ
☐	
☐	
☐	
☐	
☐	
☐	
☐	
☐	
☐	
☐	

ᦉ Stressful Thoughts ᦉ

Date: Time:

To do list	Creative Ideas
☐	
☐	
☐	
☐	
☐	
☐	
☐	
☐	
☐	
☐	

Stressful Thoughts

Date: Time:

To do list	*Creative Ideas*
☐	
☐	
☐	
☐	
☐	
☐	
☐	
☐	
☐	
☐	

Stressful Thoughts

Date:

Time:

To do list

□

□

□

□

□

□

□

□

□

□

∽ Creative Ideas ∾

∽ Stressful Thoughts ∾

Date: _____   Time: _____

To do list	Creative Ideas
☐	_____
	_____
☐	_____
	_____
☐	_____
	_____
☐	_____
	_____
☐	_____
	_____
☐	_____
	_____
☐	_____
	_____
☐	_____
	_____
☐	_____
	_____
☐	_____

Stressful Thoughts

_____

_____

_____

_____

_____

_____

Date: Time:

To do list	~ Creative Ideas ~
☐	
☐	
☐	
☐	
☐	
☐	
☐	
☐	
☐	
☐	

~ Stressful Thoughts ~

To do list

☐

☐

☐

☐

☐

☐

☐

☐

☐

☐

∾ Creative Ideas ∾

∾ Stressful Thoughts ∾

Date: Time:

To do list

Creative Ideas

☐

☐

☐

☐

☐

☐

☐

☐

☐

☐

Stressful Thoughts

Date: Time:

To do list	Creative Ideas
☐	
☐	
☐	
☐	
☐	
☐	
☐	
☐	
☐	
☐	

Stressful Thoughts

If you enjoyed this Journal please
take a moment to write a review.
Sharing your thoughts with others
greatly helps this book get into the
hands of new readers.

Thank you.

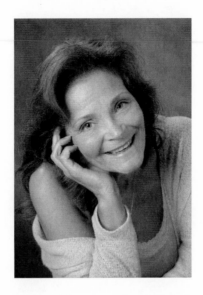

Photo by Master Photographer Jill A. Bochicchio

Author T. S. Thompson is the mother of two sons currently
living in Pennsylvania. She has a deep desire to move readers
with her books and share the light of God through them.
Thompson has been blessed with the gift of storytelling and
believes the world is in need of good family-friendly books
everyone can enjoy.

Connect with T. S. Thompson

www.ts-thompson.com

Made in United States
North Haven, CT
21 February 2022

16310351R00071